What Is Epilepsy?

A simple explanation of a complex diagnosis

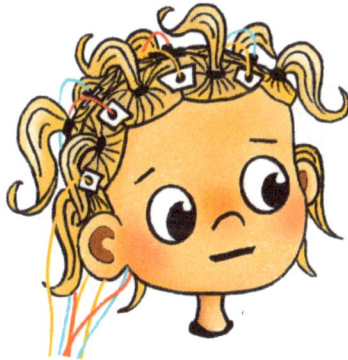

Written by Hailey Adkisson
Illustrated by Kelsey Diaz

For Juniper, my sparkly purple unicorn.
I promise to never stop fighting and advocating
for you or your beautiful purple friends.
Mommy loves you, sweet girl.

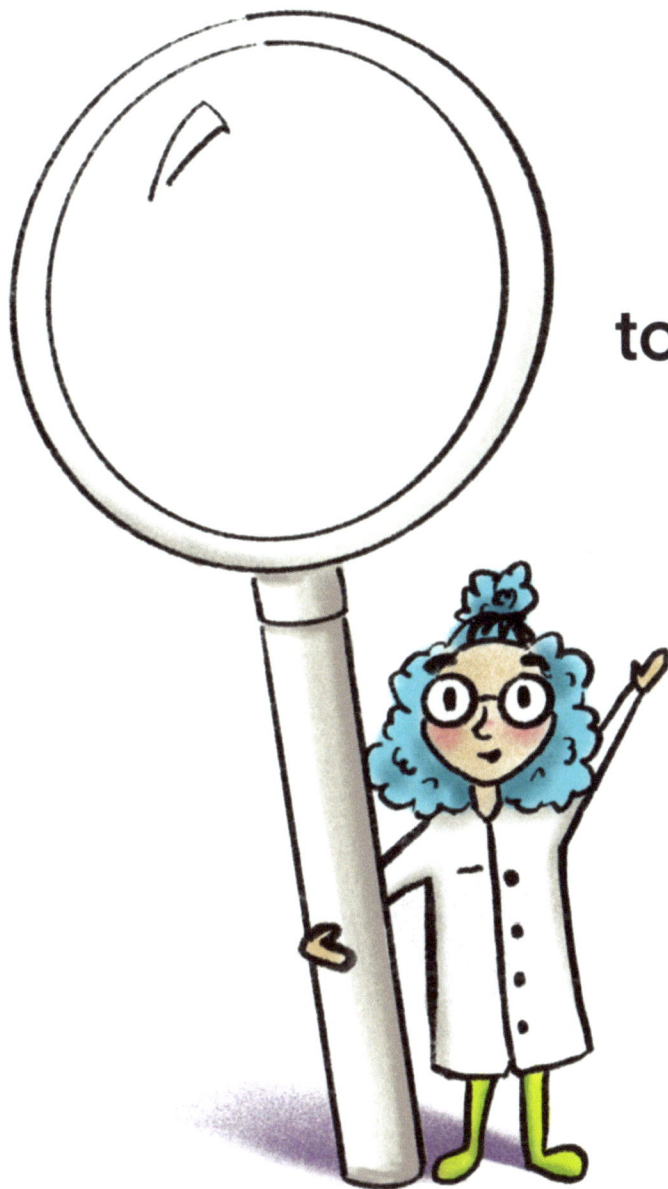

Hi! I'm Effie and today we are going to learn about epilepsy.

Did you know that your brain is electric?

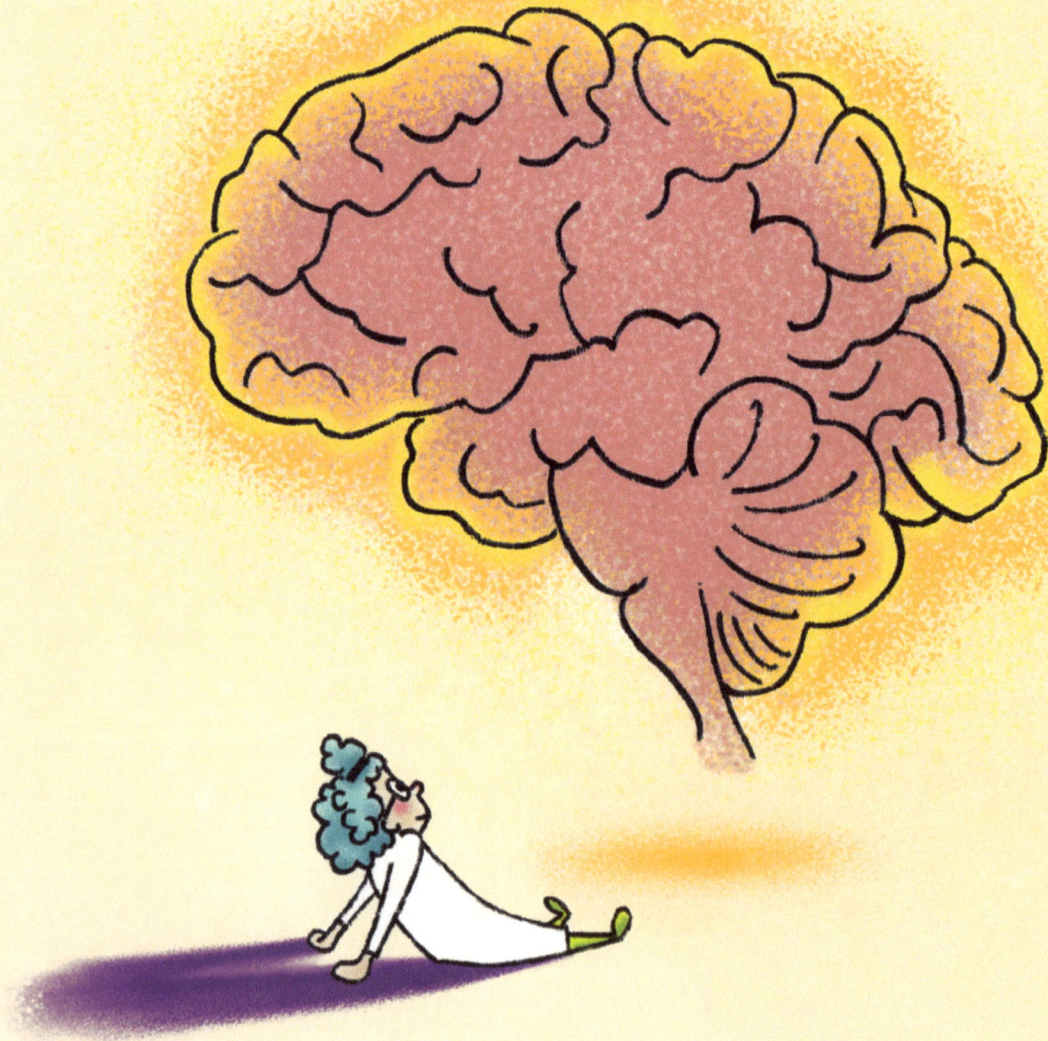

While this type of electricity can't power a lightbulb or a TV, it does power your brain and sends messages to your entire body.

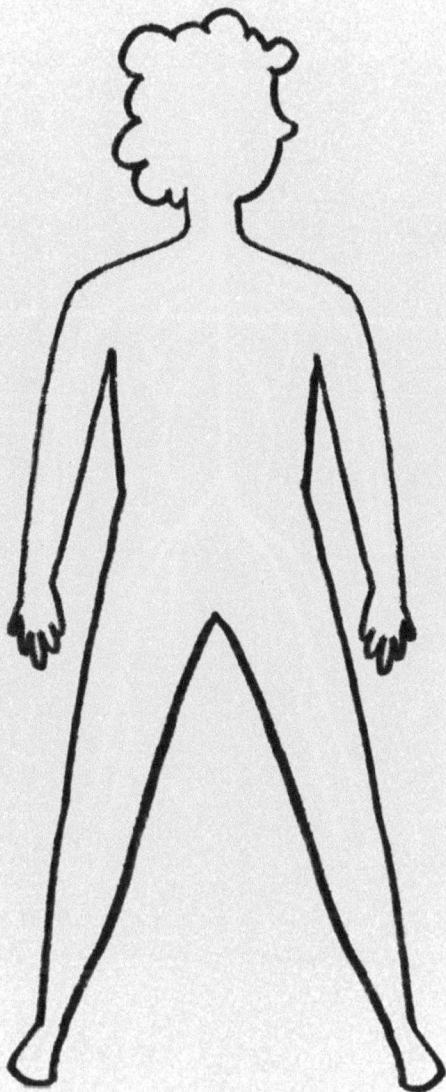

It's how we learn and grow!

But in some people, the electric activity in their brains becomes stormy and chaotic, causing a seizure.

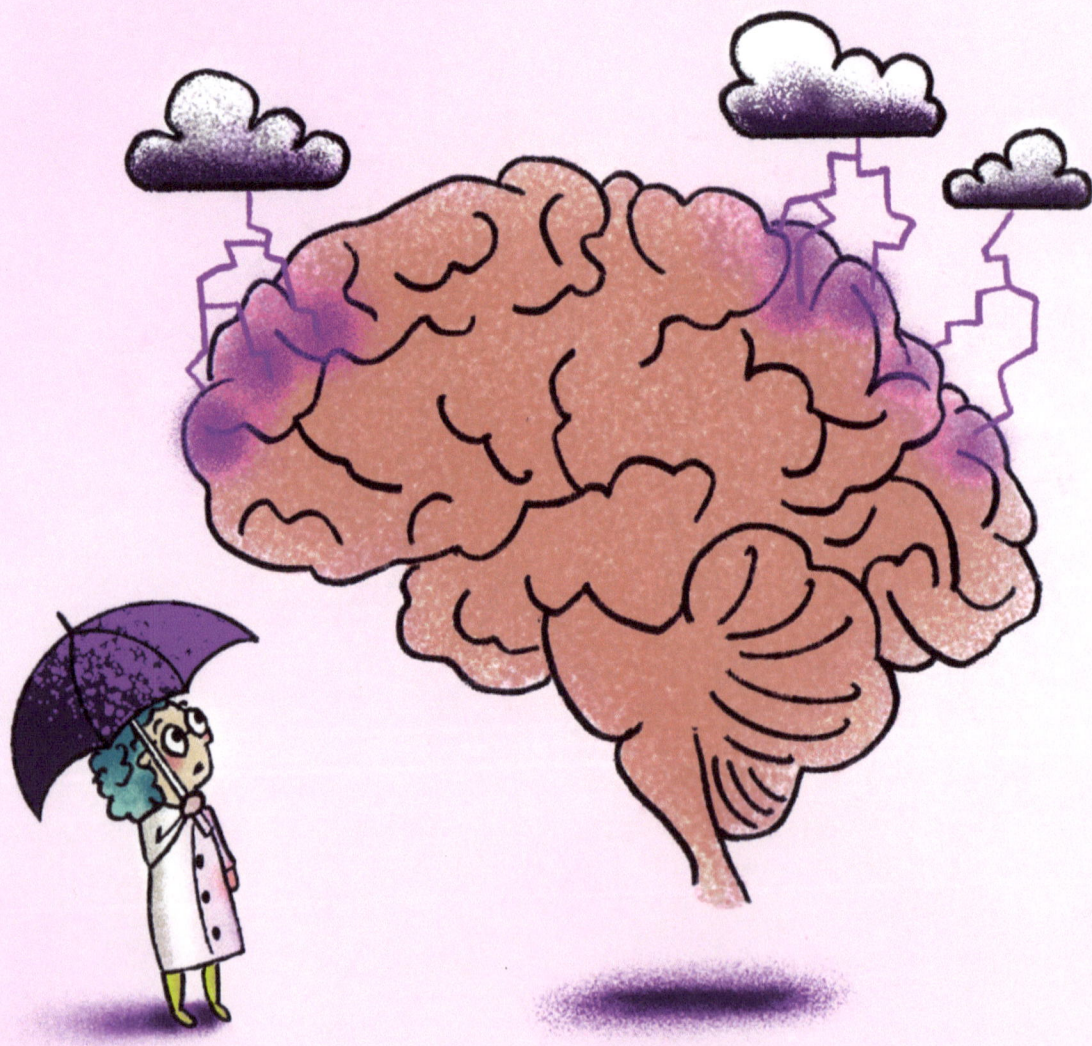

People who have many seizures have a medical condition known as epilepsy.

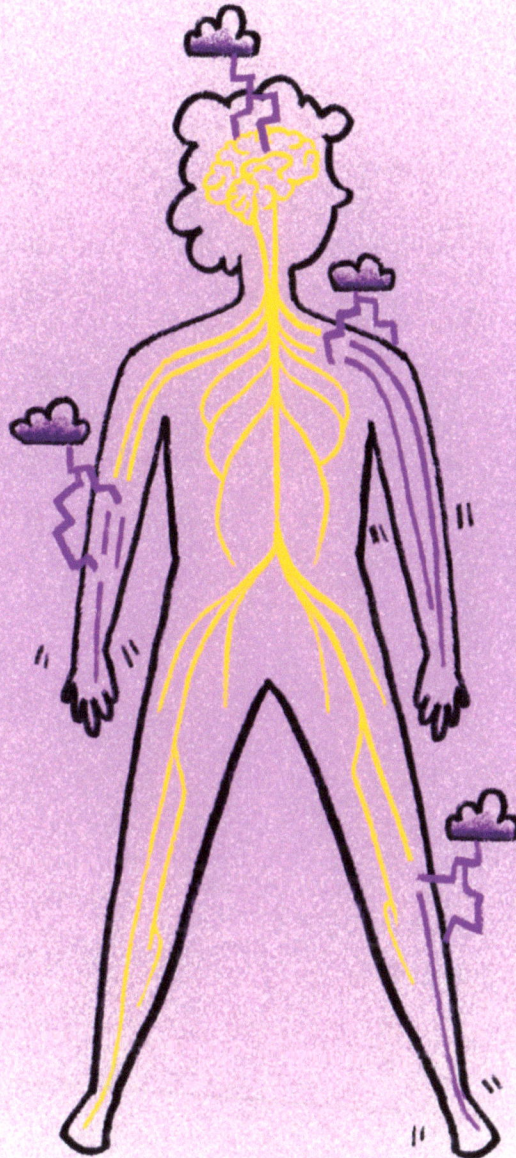

How does someone know they have epilepsy?

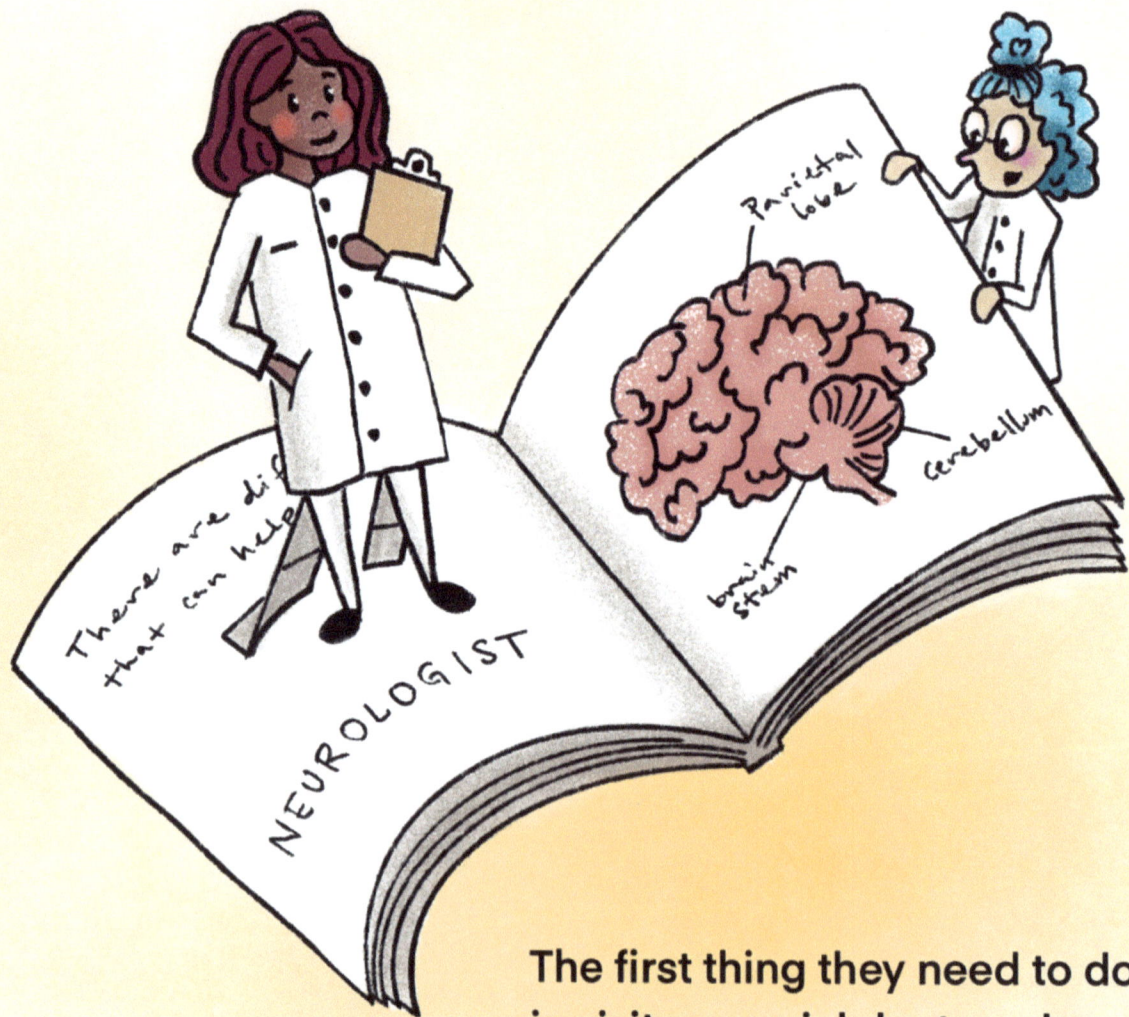

There are di[f...]
that can hel[p...]

NEUROLOGIST

Parietal lobe

cerebellum

brain stem

The first thing they need to do is visit a special doctor who studies the brain. This doctor is called a neurologist.

A neurologist can look at pictures of the brain and run other tests to see how it's working.

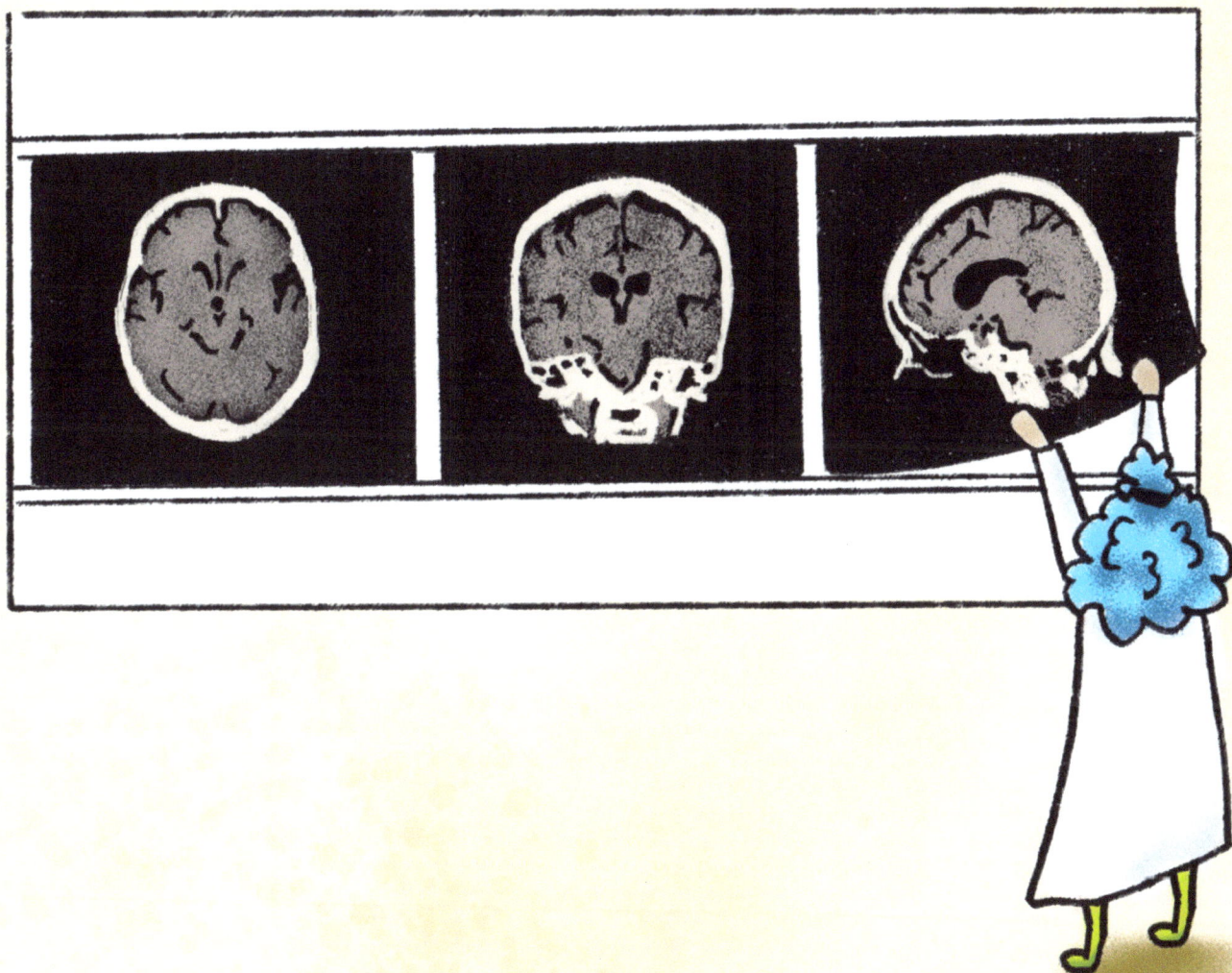

The neurologist will put stickers with wires all over the person's head. This is called an EEG. While getting an EEG may look a little silly, it doesn't hurt.

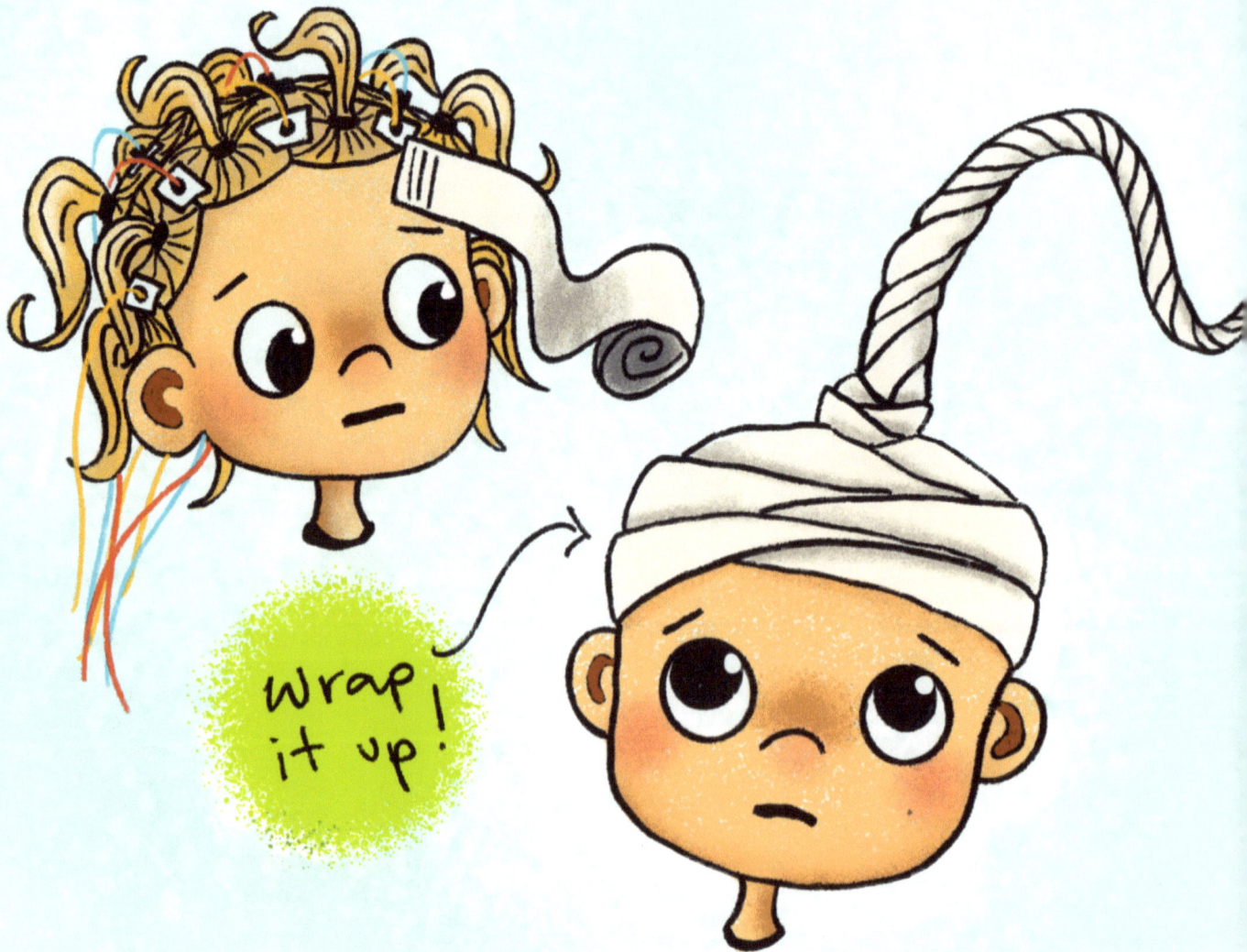

Wrap it up!

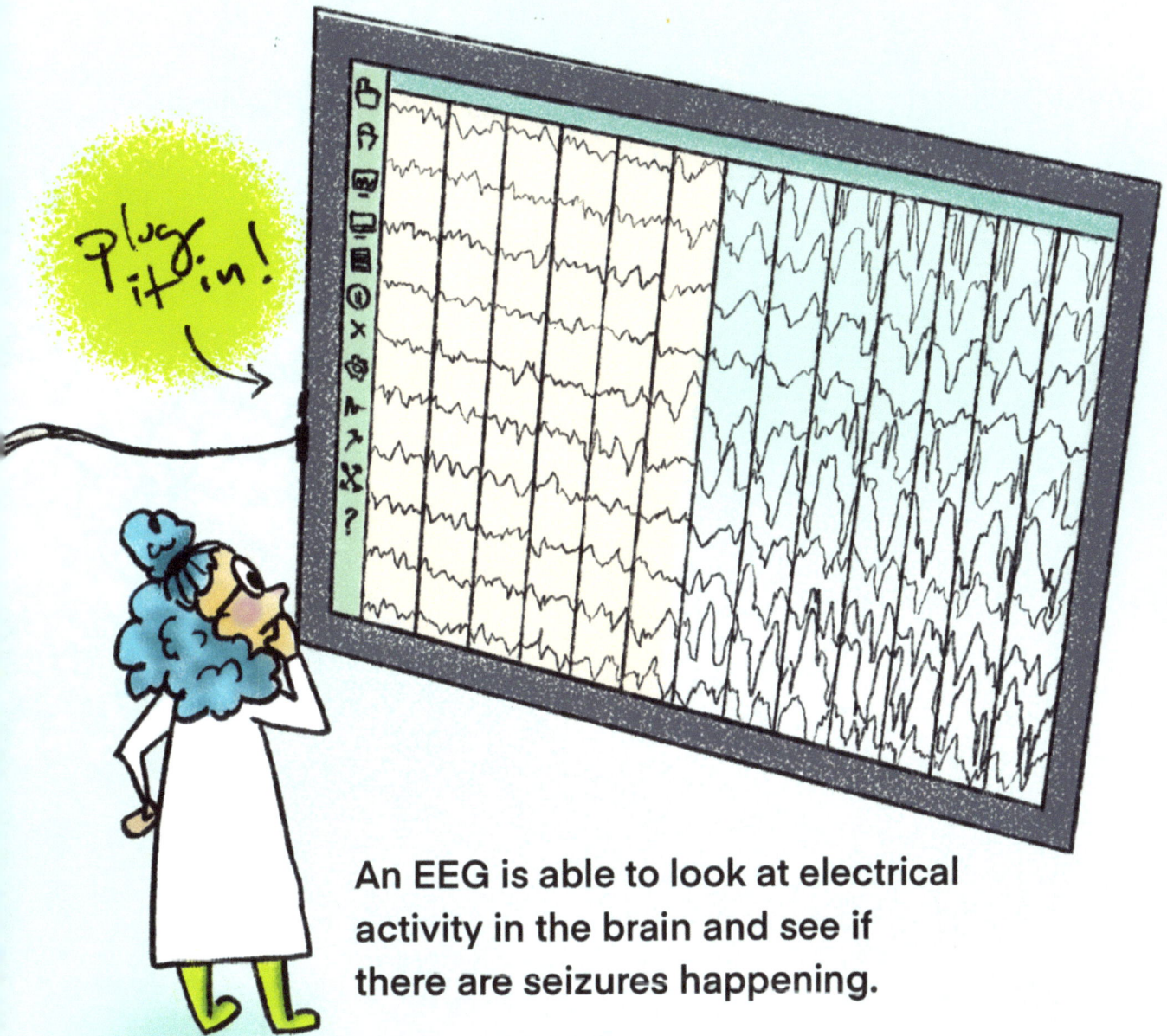

Plug it in!

An EEG is able to look at electrical activity in the brain and see if there are seizures happening.

People with no seizure activity have calm lines on their EEG . People with epilepsy often have spiky lines on their EEG.

Just like everyone looks and acts differently, seizures can look and act differently too.

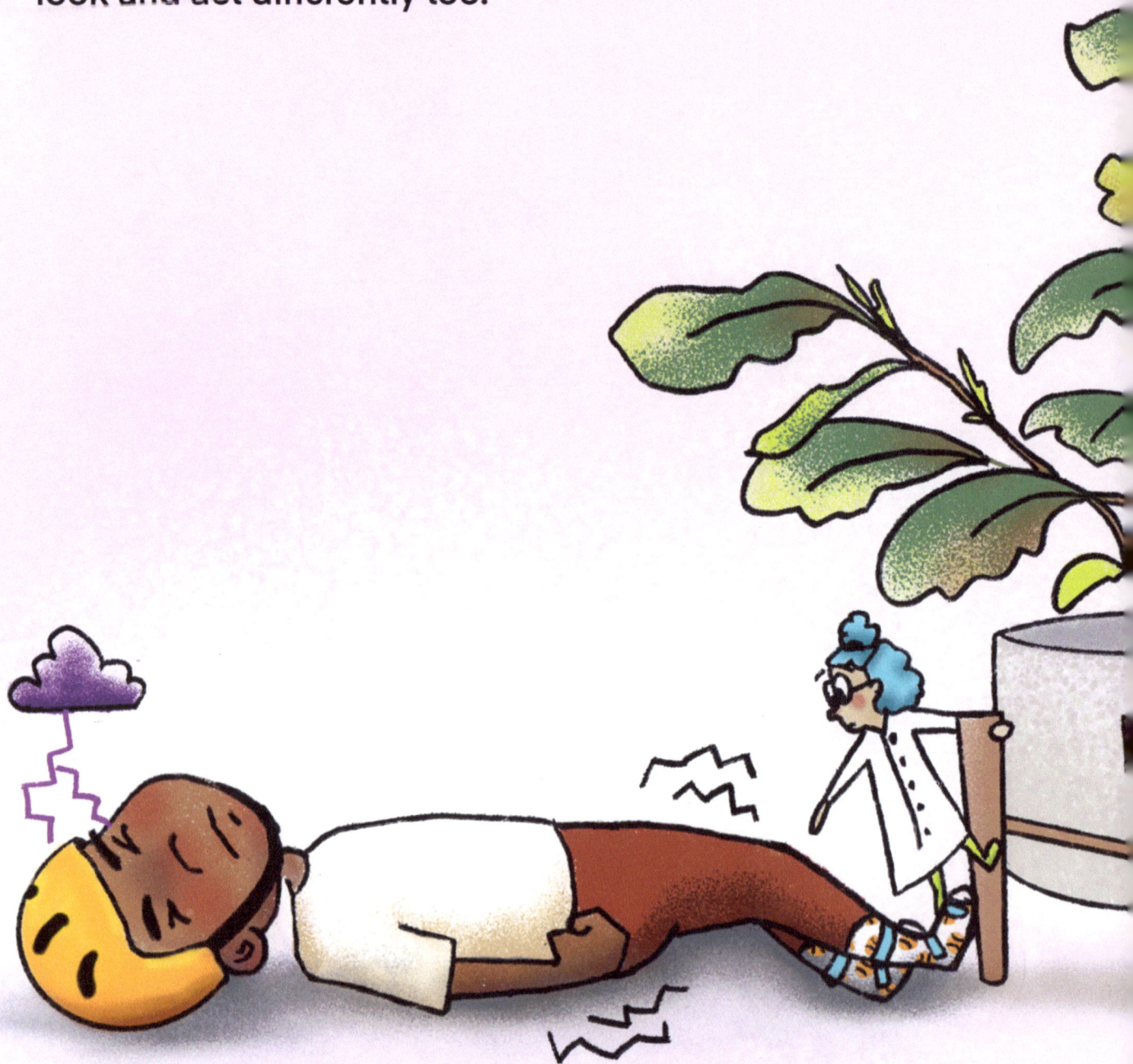

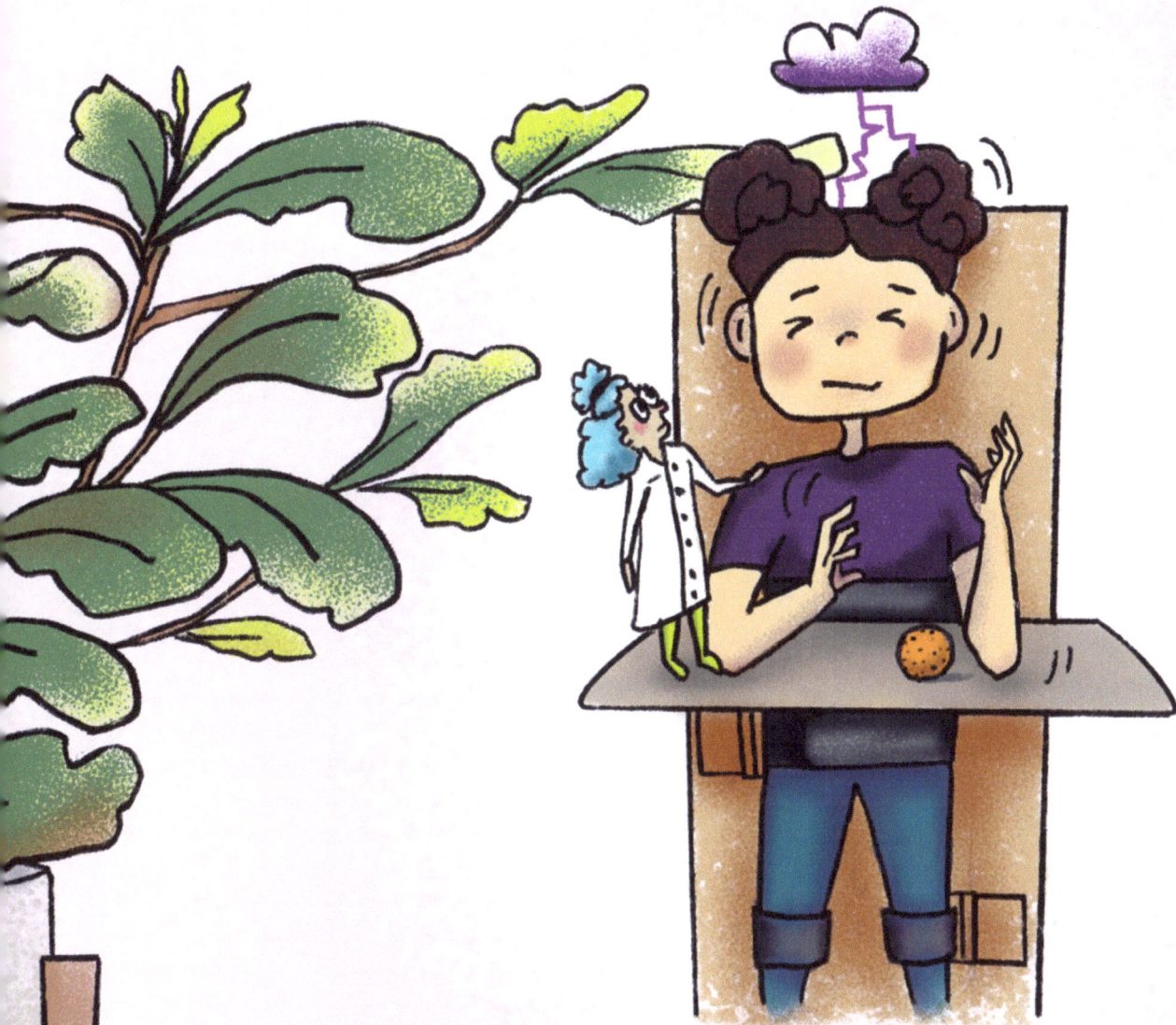

Some seizures make people shake or twitch. Other seizures can make people fall down. If someone is at risk for falling during a seizure, they may wear a helmet so they don't hurt their head.

Some seizures cause people to look like they're daydreaming. Other seizures may cause people to look like they're scared.

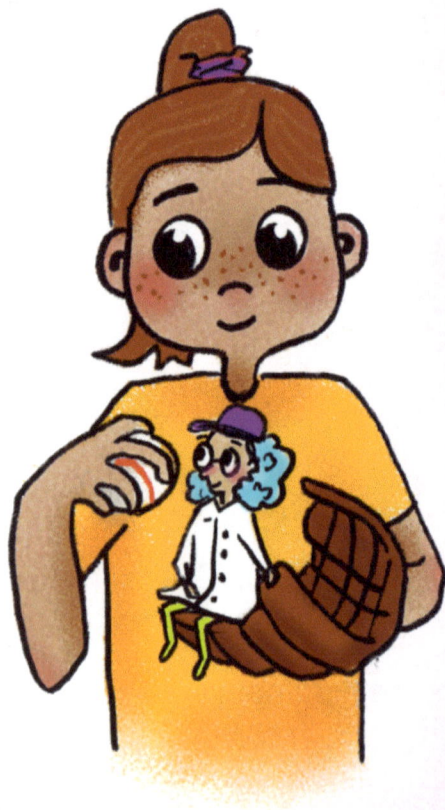

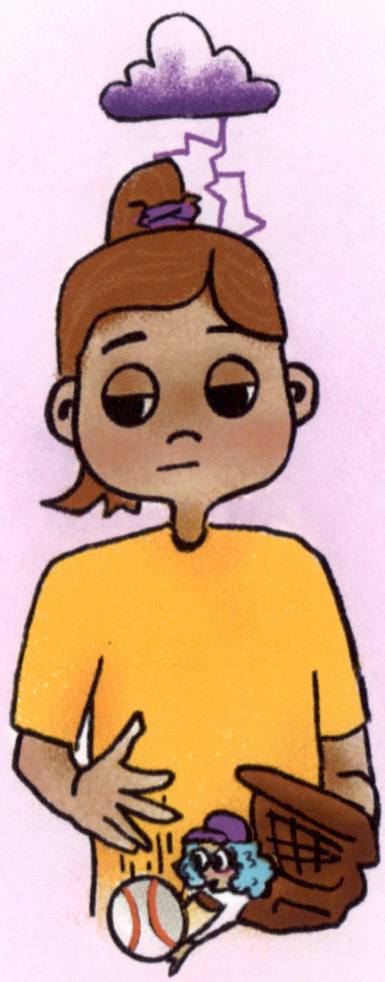

Some people get very tired after a seizure. Other people can start playing again as soon as the seizure is done.

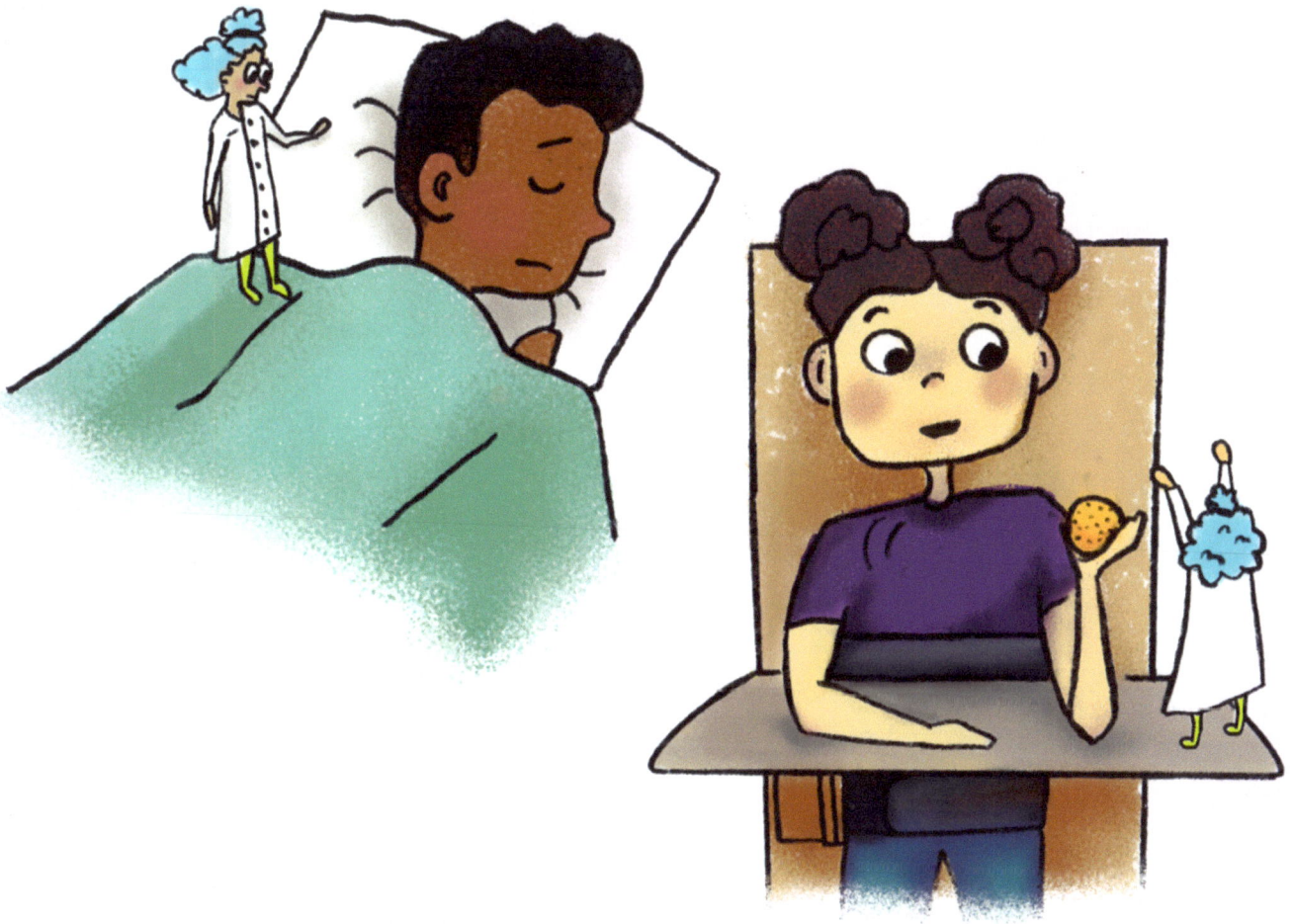

There are many different reasons people can have epilepsy.

Their brains may be smoother...

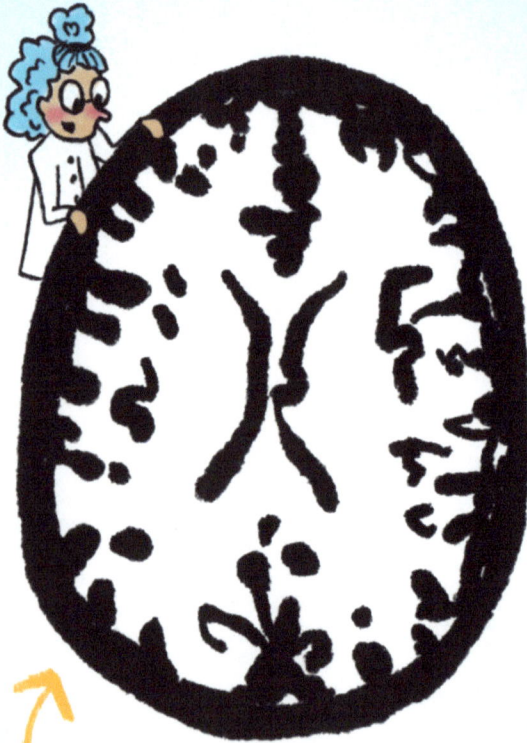

TYPICAL
BRAIN STRUCTURE

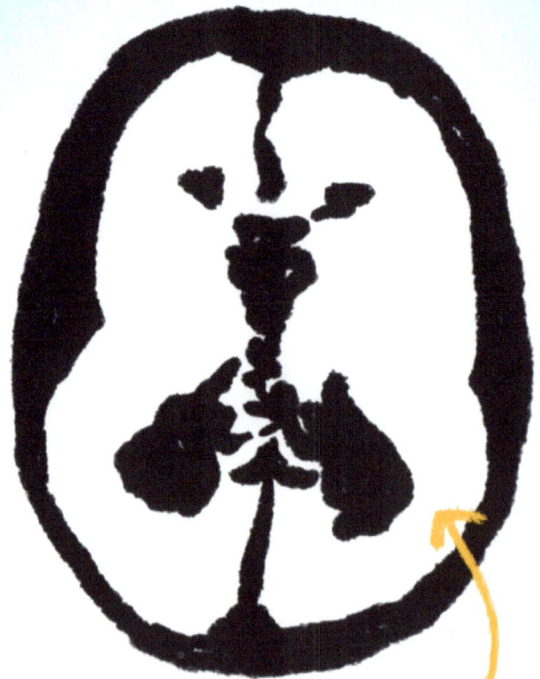

LISSENCEPHALY
or
PACHYGYRIA

We all look different from one another on the outside, and some people have brains that look different on the inside. These brain differences can cause epilepsy.

or bumpier...

or have spots on them like freckles or birthmarks.

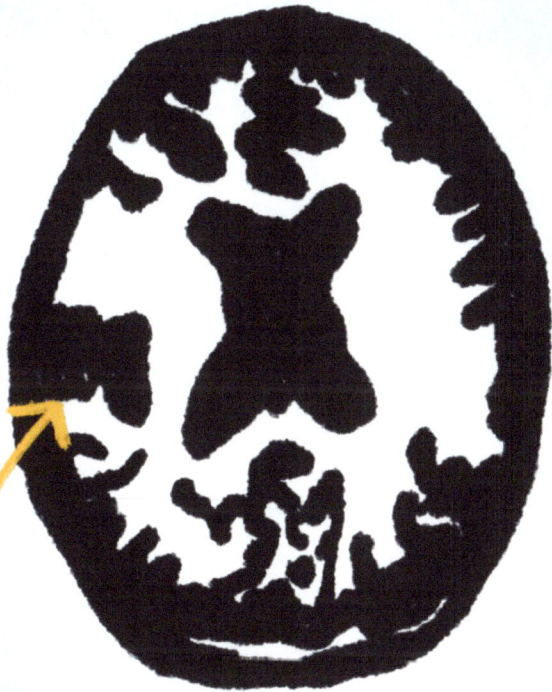

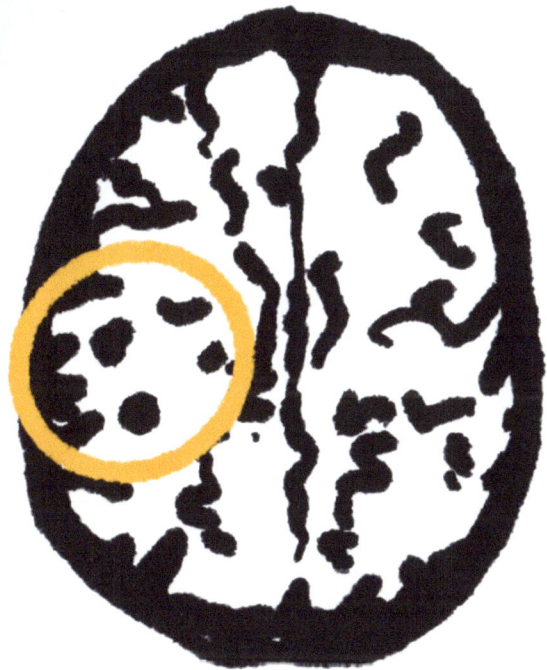

POLYMICROGYRIA

CORTICAL DYSPLASIA

Another reason someone can have epilepsy is a change in their genes.

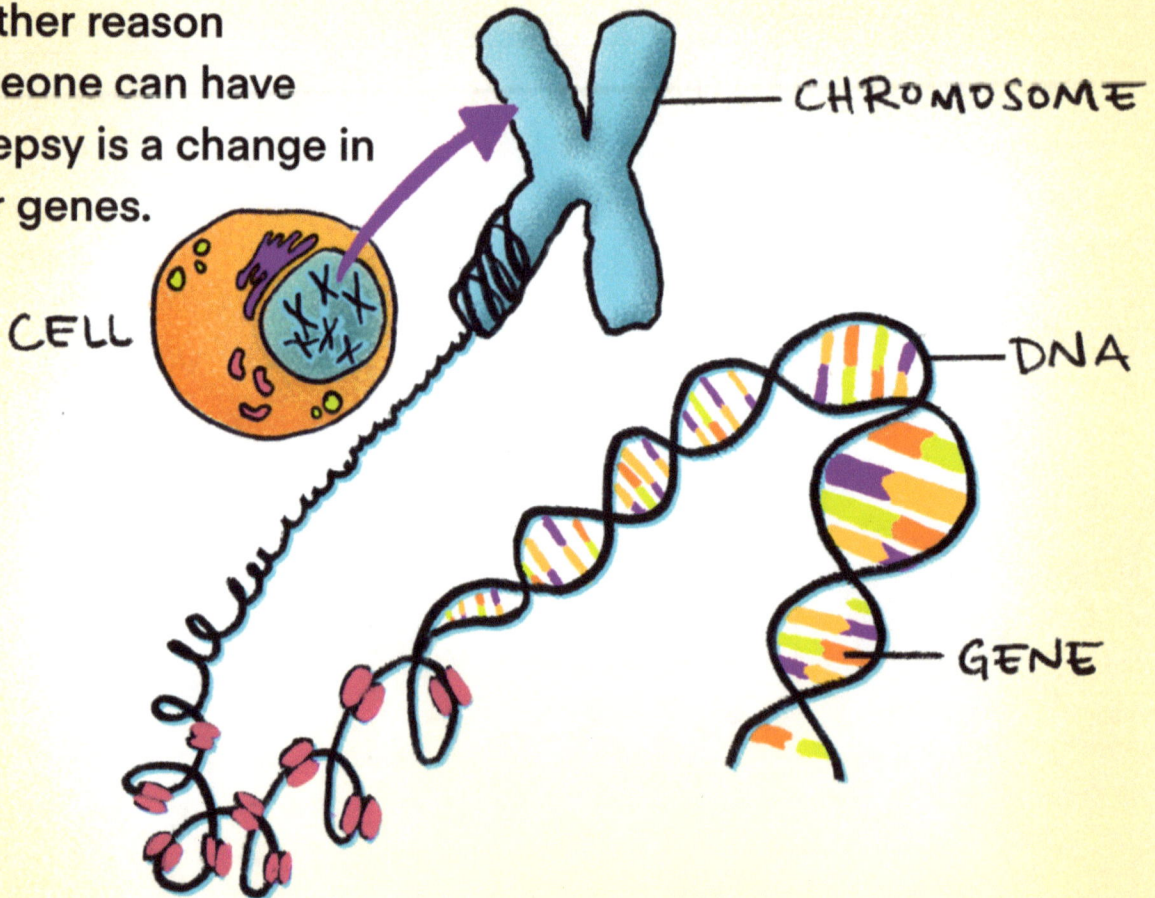

CELL

CHROMOSOME

DNA

GENE

While J-E-A-N-S are pants you wear, G-E-N-E-S are like a set of instructions that helped make you YOU when you were a little baby growing inside a tummy.

Genes decide what eye color we will have, what hair color we will have, and even how tall we will be. In some people, their genes can cause epilepsy.

Other people have epilepsy because their brain got hurt. This is called a "traumatic brain injury" or a TBI. A TBI can happen when you are being born or if you hit your head very hard.

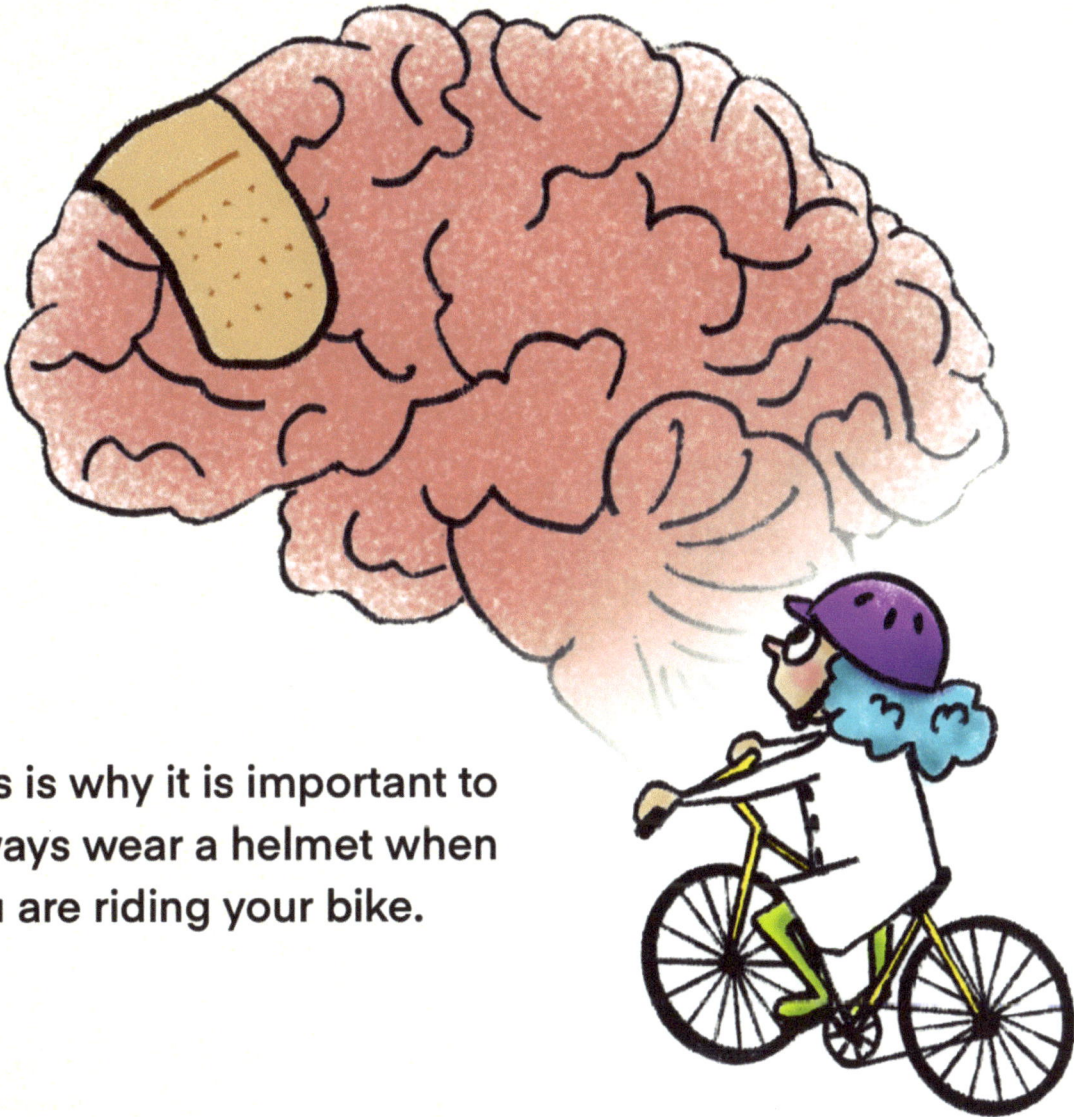

This is why it is important to always wear a helmet when you are riding your bike.

No matter the reason for someone's epilepsy, it is always very important to try and stop seizures from happening. There are many different ways neurologists work to try and do this.

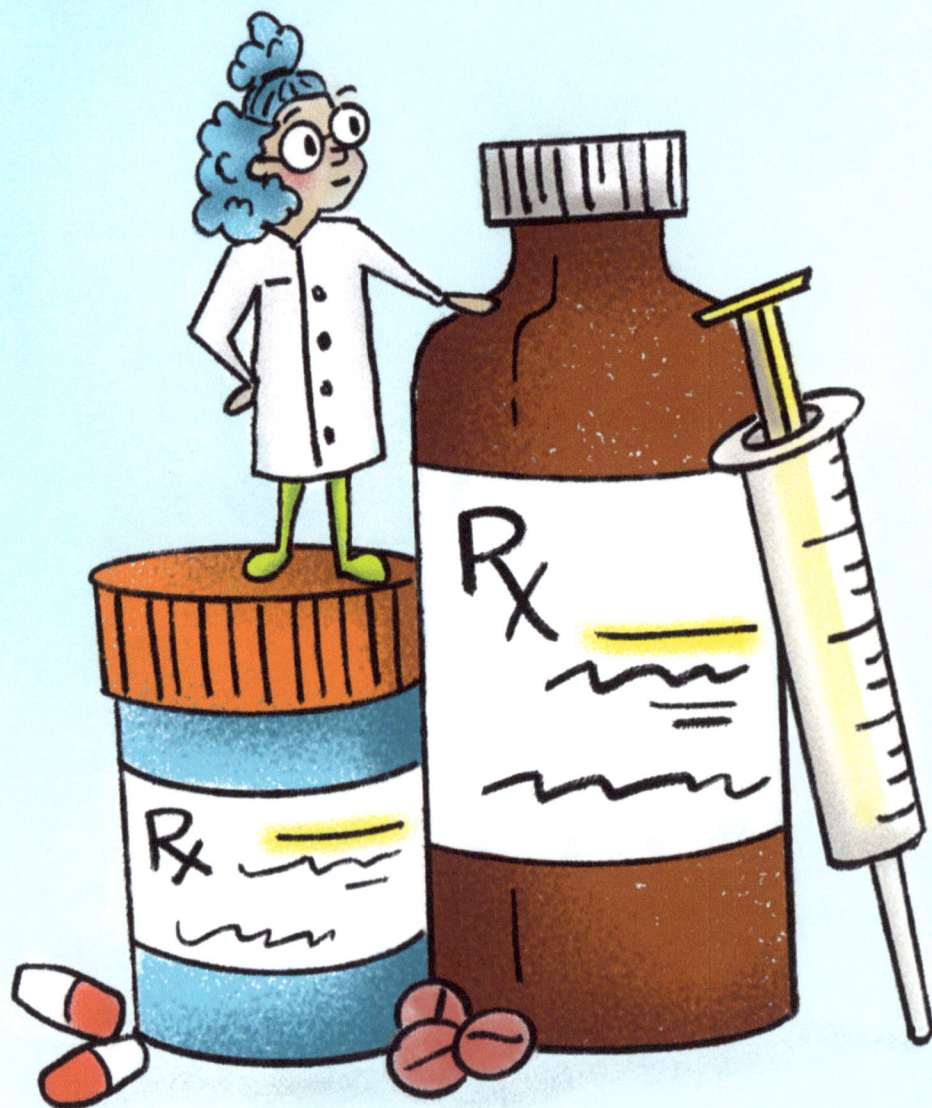

Some seizures can be stopped with medication.

Other seizures can be stopped with brain surgery.

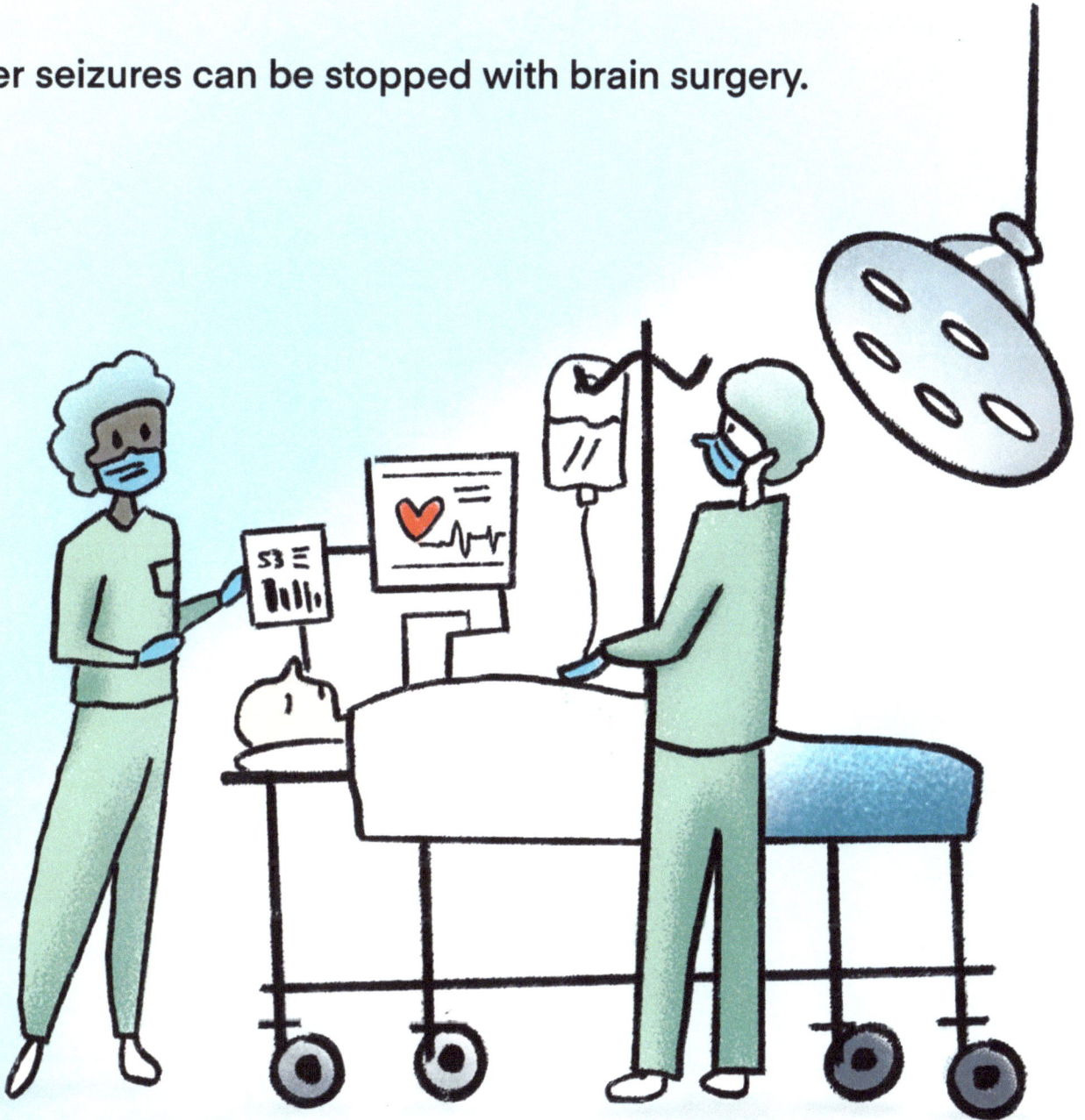

Some seizures can be stopped by eating certain foods called a medical ketogenic diet!

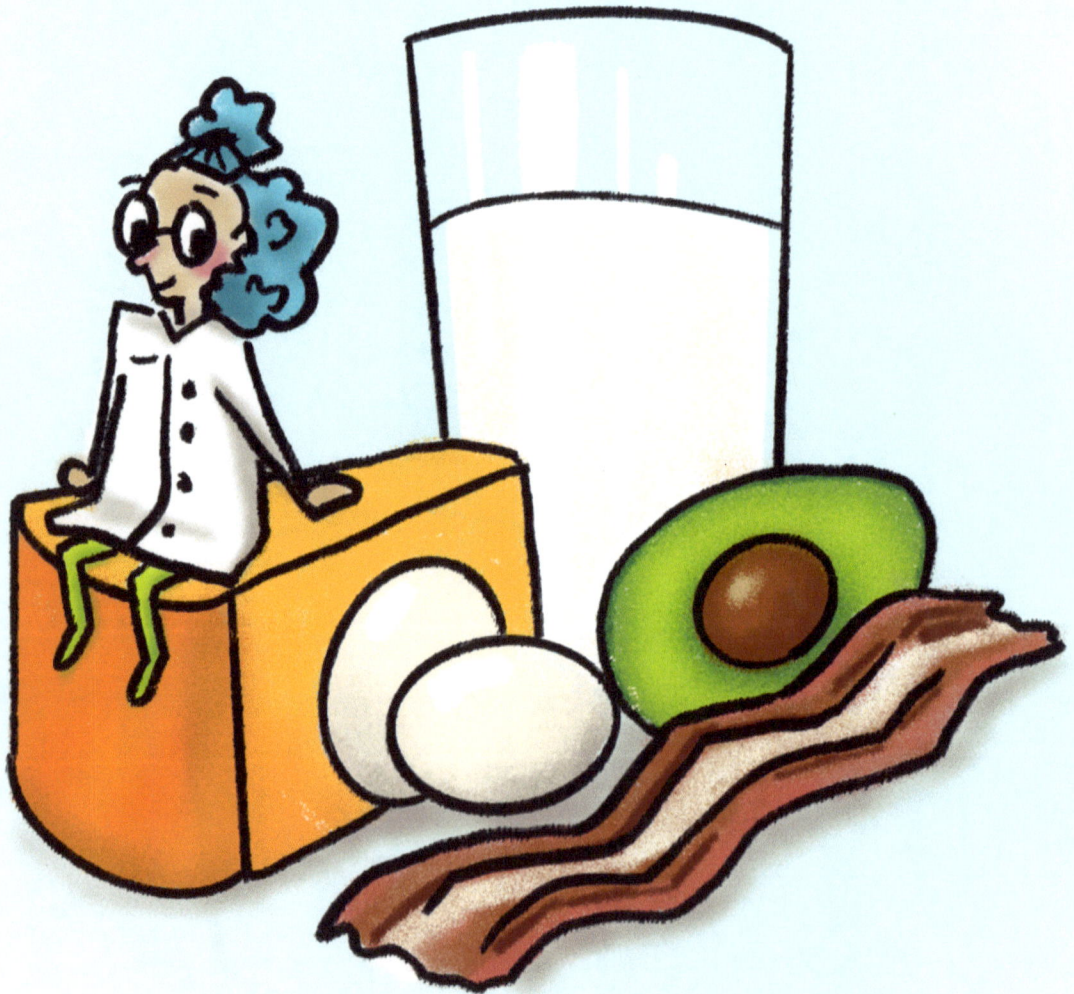

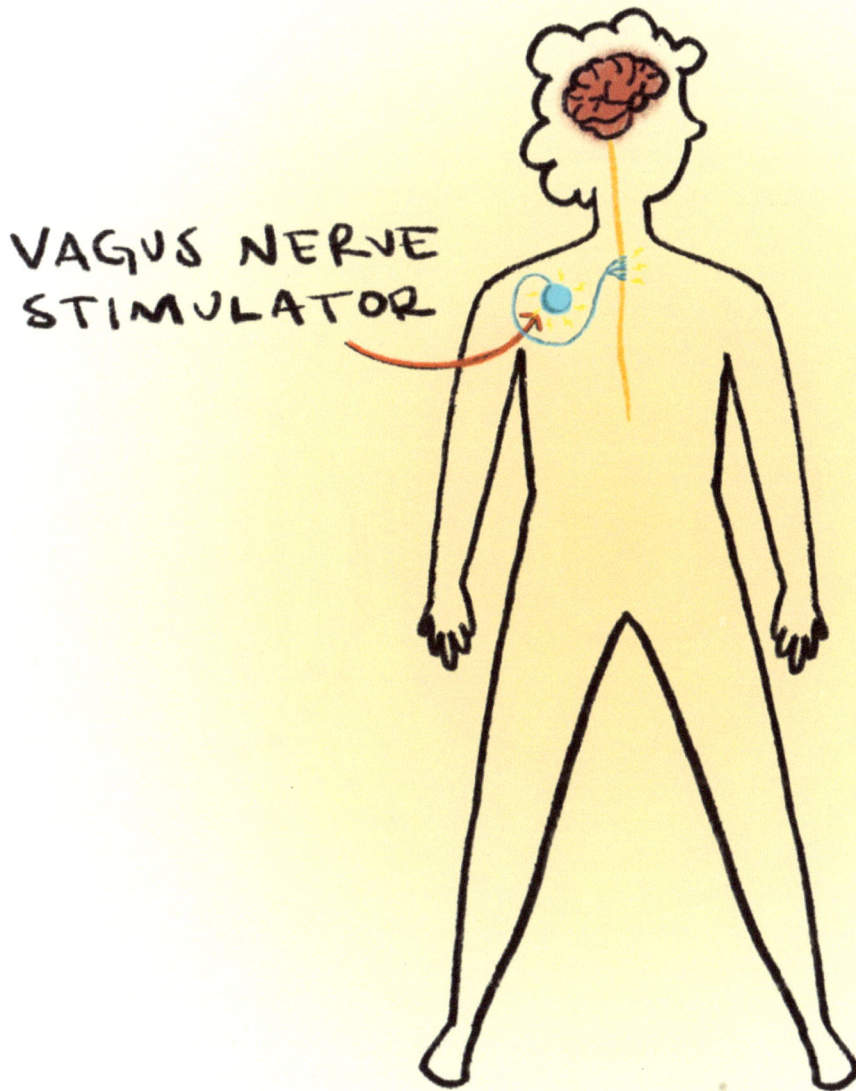

VAGUS NERVE STIMULATOR

There are even small machines that can be put inside the body to help stop and prevent seizures.

Sometimes, nothing works to stop seizures. This is called "refractory epilepsy". Refractory means something is difficult to control or stop.

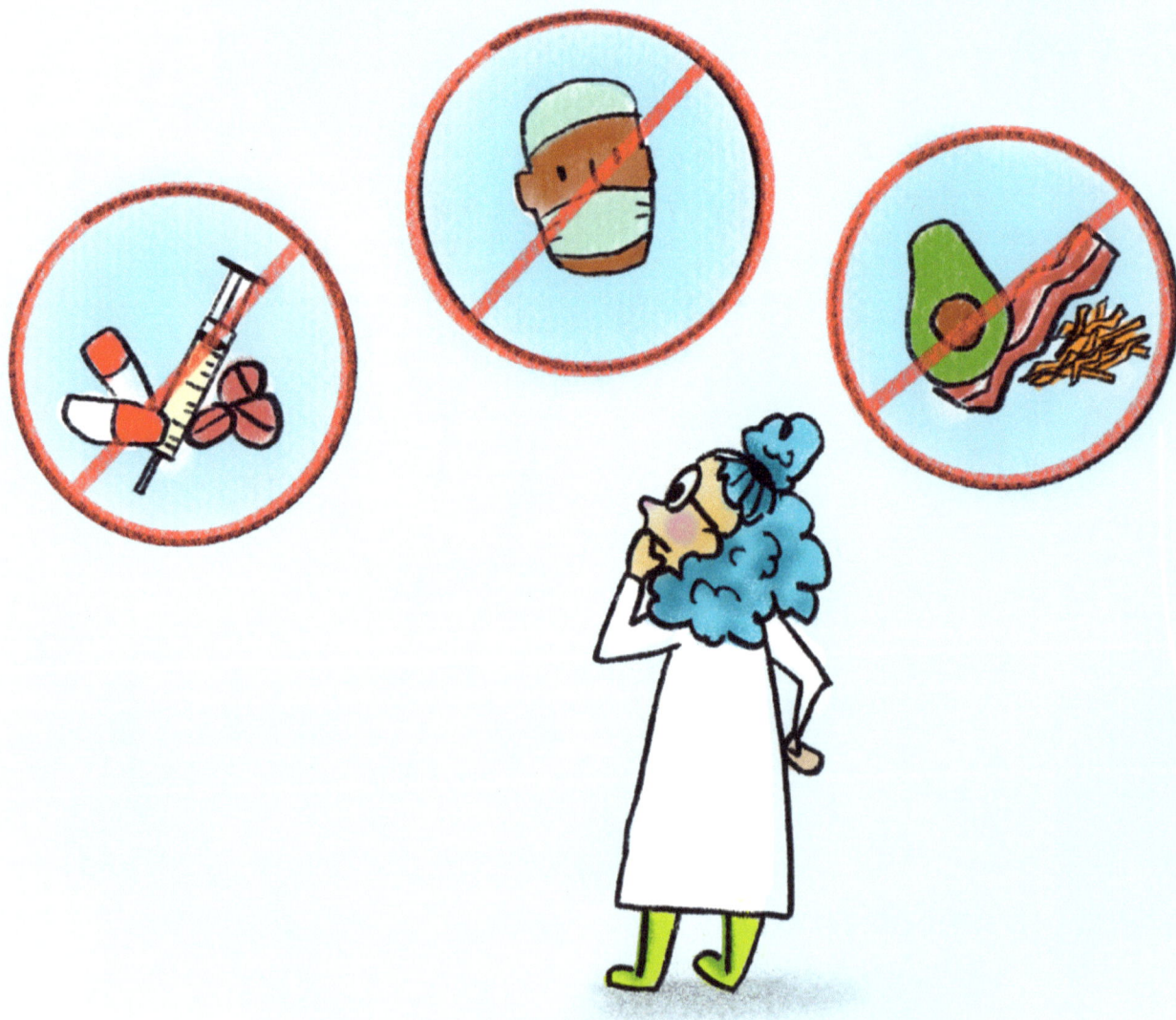

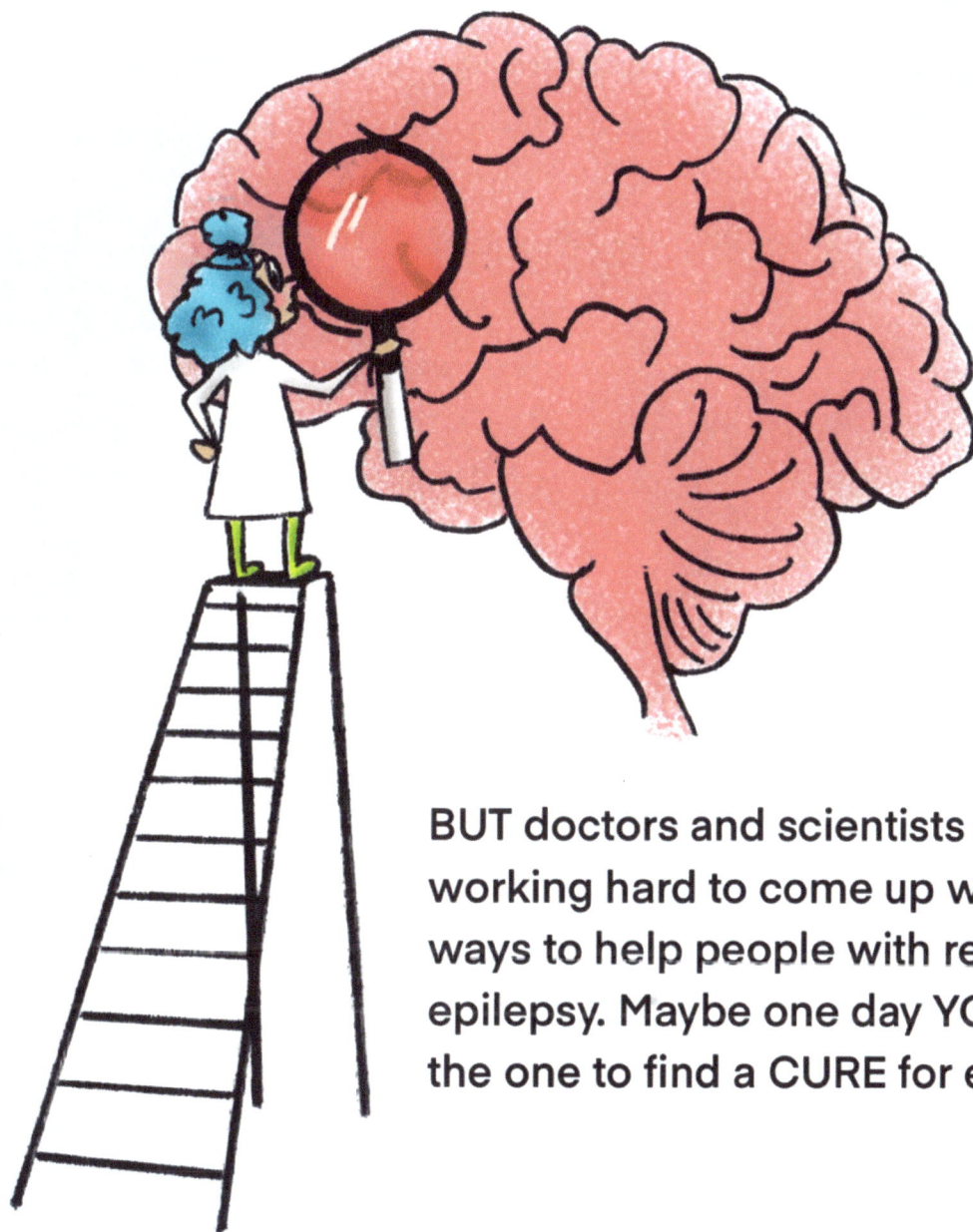

BUT doctors and scientists are working hard to come up with new ways to help people with refractory epilepsy. Maybe one day YOU can be the one to find a CURE for epilepsy!

It is important to know that epilepsy is not contagious. This means you can't catch it like you can catch a cold or the flu.

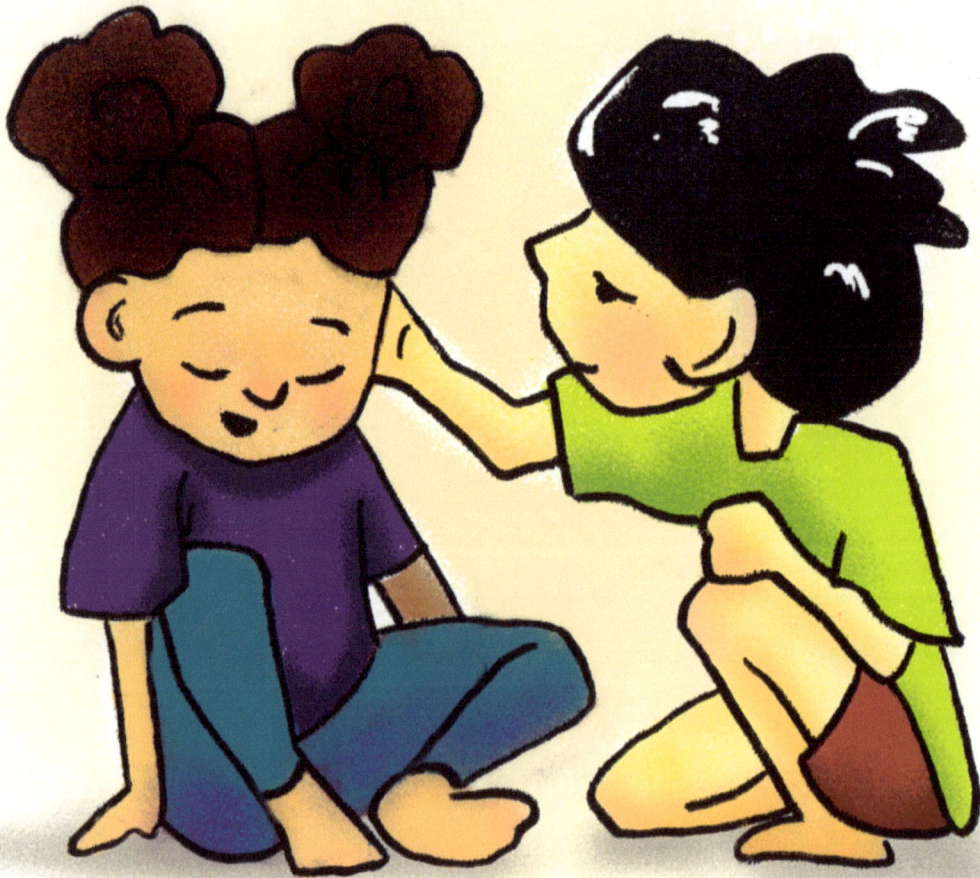

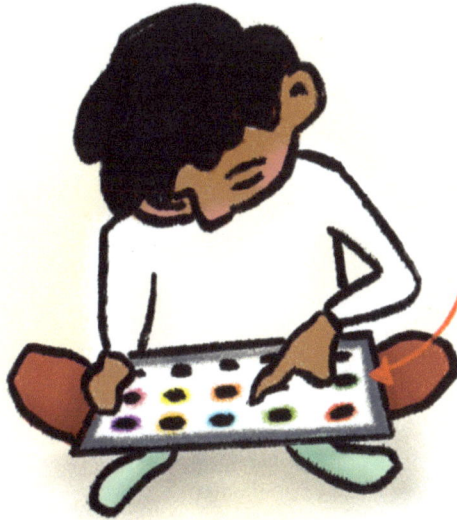

COMMUNICATION
DEVICE
(AAC)

GAIT
TRAINER

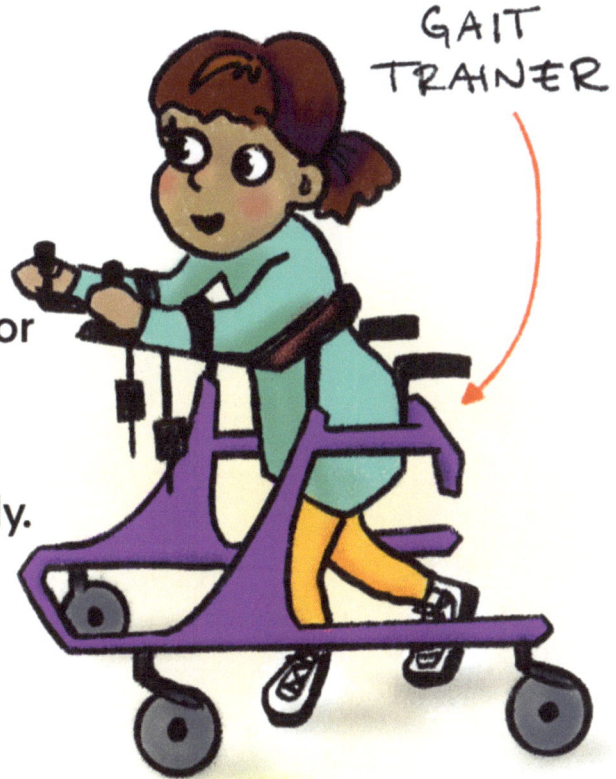

People with epilepsy may look or act different from you and me. They may move differently, talk differently, or even eat differently.

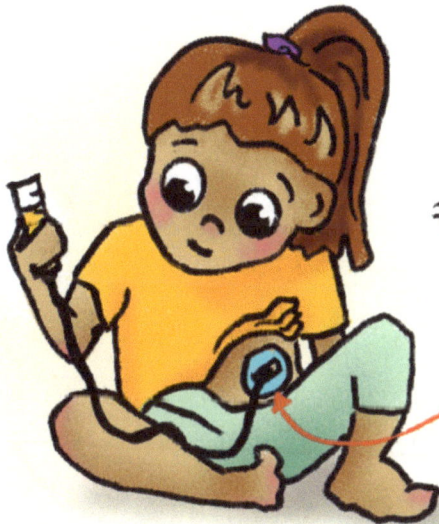

FEEDING
TUBE

But, why?

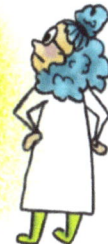

Think of epilepsy like a storm on an ocean. When there is a storm, the waves get really big. There is lightning and loud thunder. Can you imagine trying to read or do math on a boat in the middle of an ocean during a big storm? It would be very hard to learn!

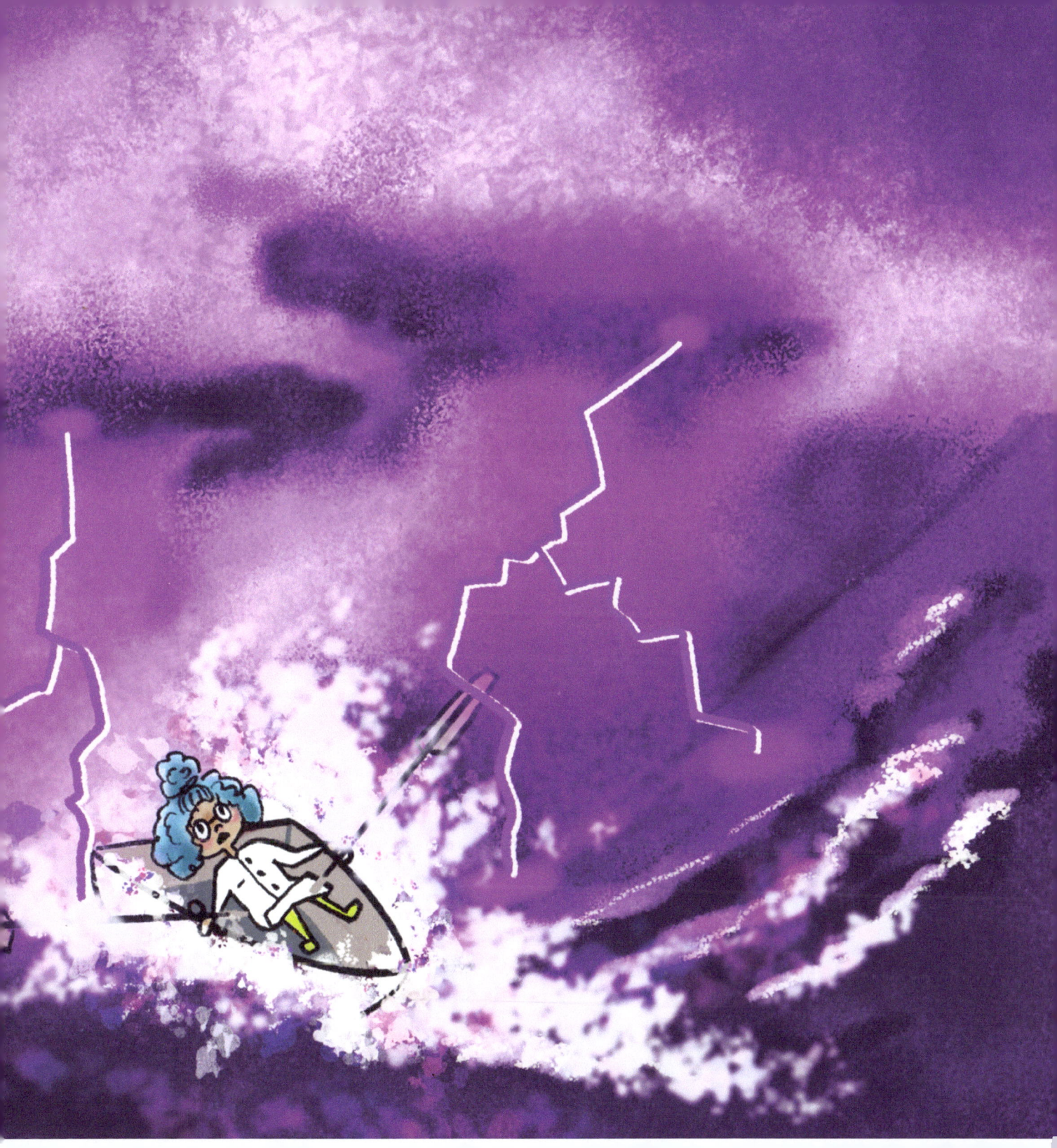

Some people with epilepsy are not able to do things that may come easily to you like walking or talking. This is because their brain has an epilepsy storm going on in it.

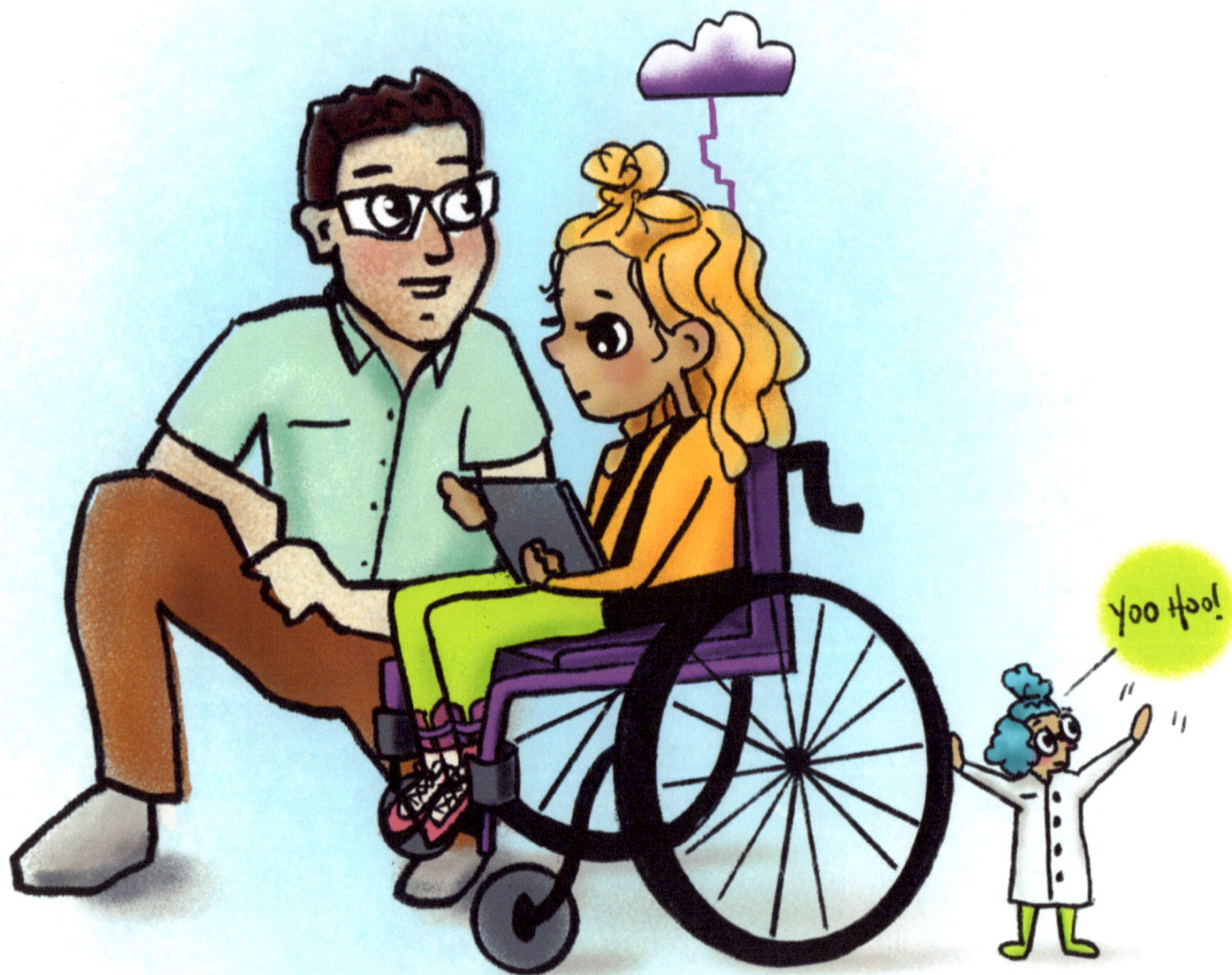

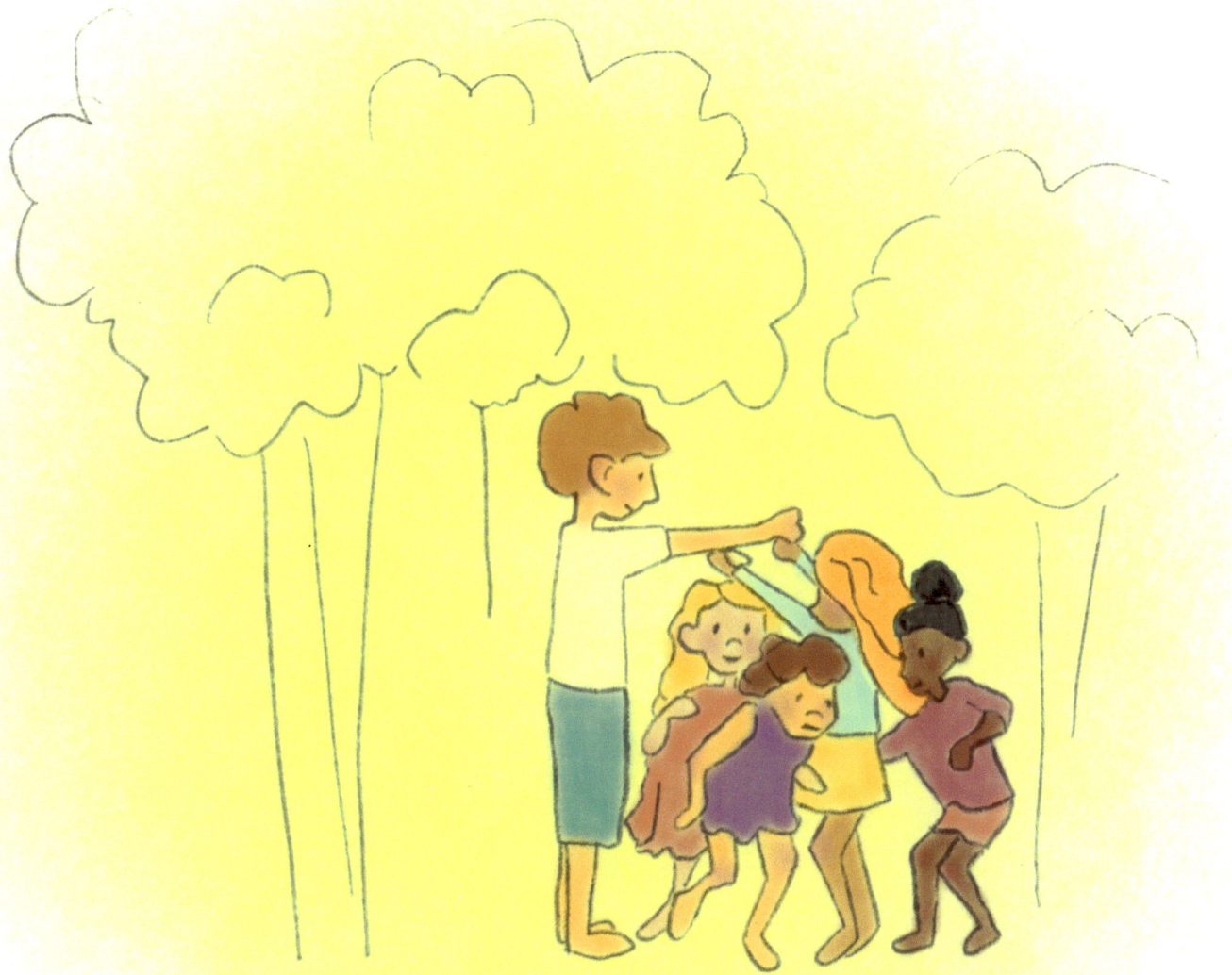

Even if someone may not be able to wave at you or play in the same way you do, they still want friends.   Instead of pointing or staring, go say "hi"! Maybe you both can make a new friend!

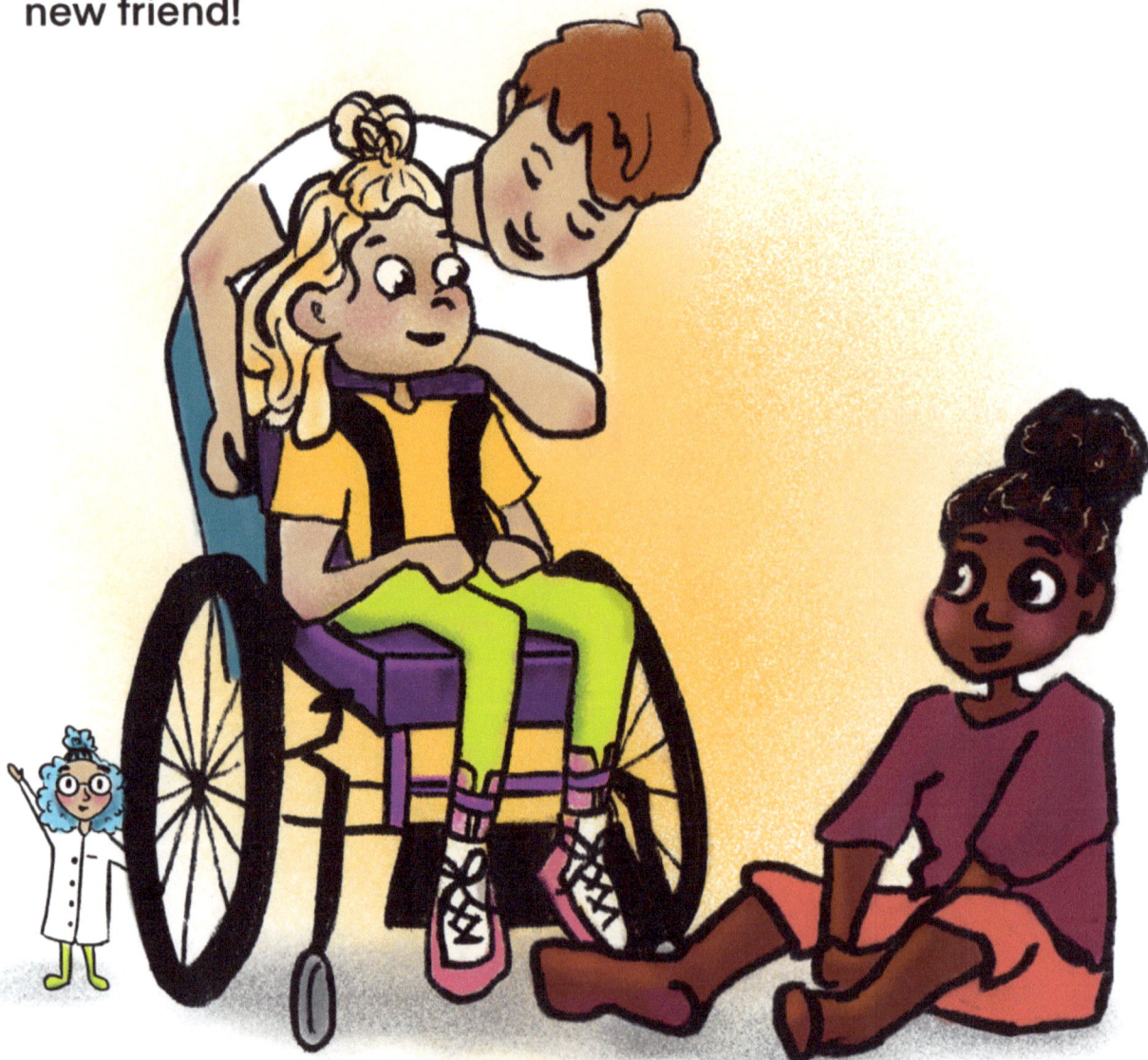

So, what should you do if you think someone is having a seizure?

✚ SEIZURE ✚ FIRST AID

☑ Step 1: Make sure they are in a SAFE place. Move away any objects that could fall or they could bump into.

☐ Step 2: Find an adult or call 9-1-1

☐ Step 3: Do not hold them down or put anything in their mouth.

☐ Step 4: STAY near them until the seizure is done and help arrives.

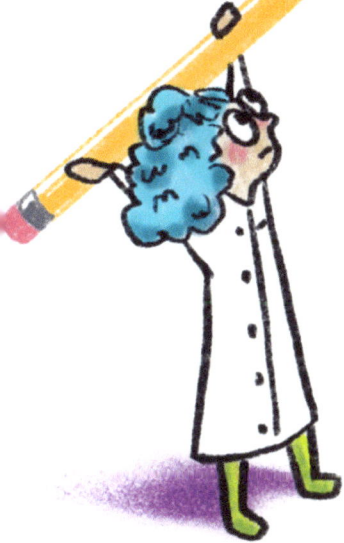

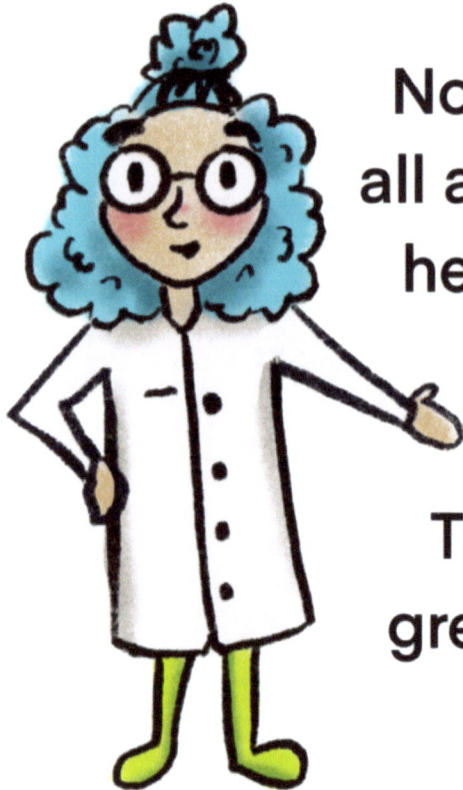

Now that you've learned
all about epilepsy, you can
help by teaching others
about it too!

Thank you for being a
great epilepsy advocate!

Appendix

Glossary
FAQ
Resources

Glossary:

AEDs (anti-epileptic drugs): Medications used to help prevent seizures in people with epilepsy. While they are not a cure for epilepsy, they can greatly reduce the number of seizures someone has.

Brain Malformation: A condition in which the brain develops abnormally. This starts before a baby is born. It is often associated with neurological and developmental problems.

Cortical Dysplasia: A type of brain malformation where the neurons in a developing brain do not reach the area they are designated to reach. This is one of the most common causes of pediatric epilepsy.

Electroencephalography (e-LEK–tro-en-SEF-uh-LOG-rah-fee) or EEG: Commonly called an EEG, this test is used to look at electrical activity in the brain, identify seizures, and diagnose epilepsy.

Epilepsy: A brain disorder that causes recurrent seizures.

Epileptologist: A neurologist who specializes in caring for people with epilepsy.

Genetic Mutation: A change in someone's DNA. At times, this change can cause seizures. Genetic mutations can be hereditary (inherited by a parent) or de-novo (not inherited).

Ketogenic Diet: Different from the fad diet, a medical ketogenic diet is a high-fat, low-carbohydrate diet that can help control seizures in some people with epilepsy. Patients are closely monitored by registered dieticians.

Refractory epilepsy: Also known as drug-resistant epilepsy, this occurs when seizures are not controlled by medication.

Neurologist: A medical doctor that focuses on diagnosing and treating issues of the nervous system and brain.

Seizure: A sudden, uncontrolled, burst of electrical activity in the brain.

Traumatic brain injury (TBI): A sudden injury to the brain.

Frequently Asked Questions

Are there different types of seizures?
Yes! There are many different types of seizures and many different words used to describe where the seizure comes from in the brain and what it looks like. A focal onset seizure starts in one area of the brain but can spread to other areas. A generalized onset seizure does not have one specific area of the brain from which the seizure originates. There are MANY different ways to classify a seizure, but here are just a few:

Tonic: Muscles in the body become stiff
Atonic: Muscles in the body relax
Myoclonic: Short jerks in parts of the body
Clonic: Continuous jerks/shakes in parts of the body

Some of these terms can combine to form other seizure types. For example, a tonic clonic seizure (previously called a grand mal) would be when a person's muscles become stiff and they start shaking continuously.

What causes epilepsy?
There are many reasons someone may have epilepsy. These could include genetics, brain injuries, structural abnormalities, or infectious disease. In some cases, a person may not know the cause of their epilepsy. This is called idiopathic epilepsy. It is important to know that epilepsy is not contagious.

Can you cure epilepsy?
At this time, there is no cure for epilepsy. However, anti-epileptic drugs (AEDs) can be very effective for many people living with epilepsy. Unfortunately, AEDs don't work for everyone. It is estimated that about $\frac{1}{3}$ of people with epilepsy have or will eventually develop refractory epilepsy. In this case, a surgical evaluation can be beneficial to see if the individual is a candidate for brain surgery or implanted devices to treat epilepsy.

Are all seizures epilepsy?
No. Not all seizures are epilepsy. Epilepsy, sometimes called a "seizure disorder", is characterized by recurrent seizures, more than 24 hours apart, which have not been caused by a specific event (e.g. infection, fever, blood sugar fluctuations, etc.). If a person has more than one seizure and a probability of future seizures, they can be diagnosed with epilepsy.

How common is epilepsy?

Epilepsy is not rare. In fact, 1 in 26 people in the United States will develop epilepsy in their lifetime. Epilepsy affects more people than multiple sclerosis, cerebral palsy, Parkinson's disease, and ALS combined.

Can you outgrow epilepsy?

While some children can outgrow epilepsy, many will still require daily medication throughout their lifetime. It is important to keep in mind that not all seizures are epilepsy. While febrile seizures are common in children and can be outgrown, epilepsy is a more complex diagnosis. Epilepsy is most common among very young children or adults over the age of 65.

Is epilepsy dangerous?

Yes. Individuals diagnosed with epilepsy, especially those with refractory epilepsy, are at greater risk of death or injury due to seizures. This is why treatment and developing a seizure protocol is important. SUDEP (sudden unexplained death by epilepsy) is the leading cause of epilepsy-related death.

When is Epilepsy Awareness Month?

November is Epilepsy Awareness Month! Wear purple (the color of epilepsy awareness) and show your support for those diagnosed with epilepsy.

What should I do if I think my child is having seizures?

If you think your child is having a seizure, follow the seizure first-aid protocol. Stay with them and start timing the seizure. Keep your child safe. Make sure there is nothing around they could bump into. Roll them to their side if they are not able to do so themselves. Do not stick anything in their mouth. Record the seizure on video to be able to show medical providers. If the seizure lasts longer than five minutes, or they are having difficulty breathing, call 911. If the seizure stops without requiring calling 911, contact your child's medical team and show them the video.

If you go to a hospital, you are strongly encouraged to go to a children's hospital. If at all possible, go to a children's hospital that is considered a level 4 epilepsy center as they provide care for the most complex forms of epilepsy. Unsure what level your local children's hospital is? Search online at the National Association of Epilepsy Centers website (https://www.naec-epilepsy.org/).

References:

1. Refractory epilepsy. Hopkinsmedicine.org. Published November 19, 2019. Accessed July 3, 2023. https://www.hopkinsmedicine.org/health/conditions-and-diseases/epilepsy/refractory-epilepsy

2. Facts & statistics about epilepsy. Epilepsy Foundation. Accessed July 3, 2023. https://www.epilepsy.com/what-is-epilepsy/statistics

3. Risks associated with epilepsy. CURE Epilepsy. Published December 31, 2021. Accessed July 3, 2023. https://www.cureepilepsy.org/for-patients/understanding/basics/challenges-risks/

4. Sudden unexpected death in epilepsy (SUDEP). Cdc.gov. Published September 30, 2020. Accessed July 3, 2023. https://www.cdc.gov/epilepsy/about/sudep/index.htm

5. Committee on the Public Health Dimensions of the Epilepsies, Board on Health Sciences Policy, Institute of Medicine. Epilepsy across the Spectrum: Promoting Health and Understanding. (England MJ, Liverman CT, Schultz AM, Strawbridge LM, eds.). National Academies Press; 2012.

6. QuickStats: Age-adjusted percentages* of adults aged →18 years who have epilepsy, by epilepsy status(†) and race/ethnicity(§) - national health interview survey, United States, 2010 and 2013 combined(¶). MMWR Morb Mortal Wkly Rep. 2016;65(23):611. doi:10.15585/mmwr.mm6523a8

Want to learn more about epilepsy? Here are some great resources to check out!

Child Neurology Foundation (www.childneurologyfoundation.org)

Cure Epilepsy (www.cureepilepsy.org)

Danny Did Foundation (https://www.dannydid.org/)

DEE-P Connections (www.deepconnections.net)

Epilepsy Alliance America (www.epilepsyallianceamerica.org/)

Epilepsy Foundation (www.epilepsy.com)

Lennox-Gastaut Foundation (https://www.lgsfoundation.org/)

National Association of Epilepsy Centers (www.naec-epilepsy.org)

Pediatric Epilepsy Surgery Alliance (https://epilepsysurgeryalliance.org/)

www.ingramcontent.com/pod-product-compliance
Lightning Source LLC
Chambersburg PA
CBHW041539260326
41914CB00015B/1508